CARNIVORE DIET FOR WOMEN OVER 50

35 Easy Recipes for Weight Loss and Healthy Muscle Mass

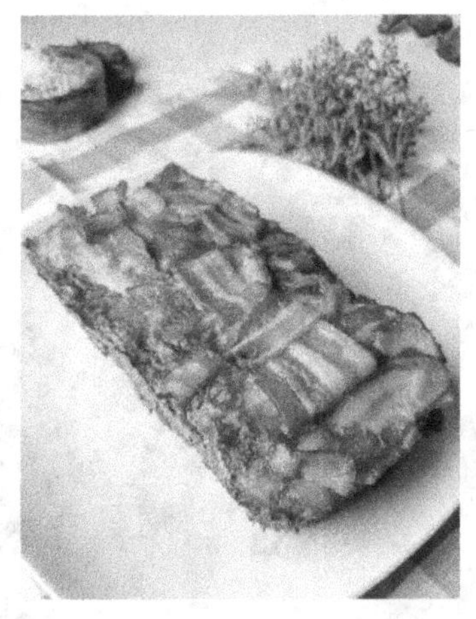

Mey W Smith

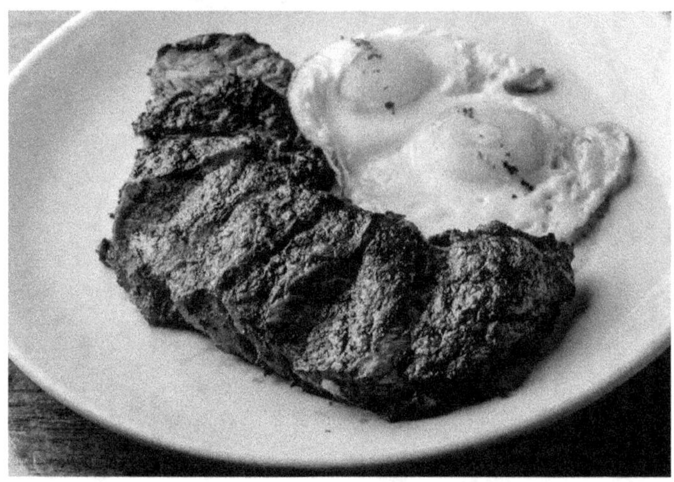

HOW TO USE THIS COOKBOOK

1. Understand the Basics: Familiarize yourself with the fundamentals of the carnivore diet, which primarily consists of consuming animal-based foods such as meat, fish, eggs, and some dairy products while avoiding plant-based foods like fruits, vegetables, grains, and legumes.

2. Plan Your Meals: Create a meal plan that includes a variety of animal-based protein sources, such as beef, poultry, seafood, and organ meats. Incorporate fats like butter, ghee, and tallow for satiety and energy. Ensure your meals are balanced and satisfying to meet your nutritional needs.

3. Stay Hydrated: Drink plenty of water to stay hydrated, especially since the carnivore diet tends to be low in carbohydrates, which can lead to increased water loss. Opt for filtered water or mineral water to replenish electrolytes and support overall hydration.

4. Listen to Your Body: Pay attention to how your body responds to the carnivore diet. Some women may experience initial adjustments, such as changes in digestion or energy levels. Be mindful of any signs of discomfort or nutrient deficiencies, and adjust your diet accordingly by incorporating supplements or consulting with a healthcare professional.

5. Monitor Your Progress: Keep track of your health and progress on the carnivore diet. Monitor factors such as weight, energy levels, mental clarity, and overall well-being. Adjust your diet as needed to optimize your results and ensure you're meeting your health goals.

By following these five easy steps, women over 50 can effectively use the carnivore diet to support their health and well-being, enjoying the benefits of a nutrient-dense, animal-based dietary approach.

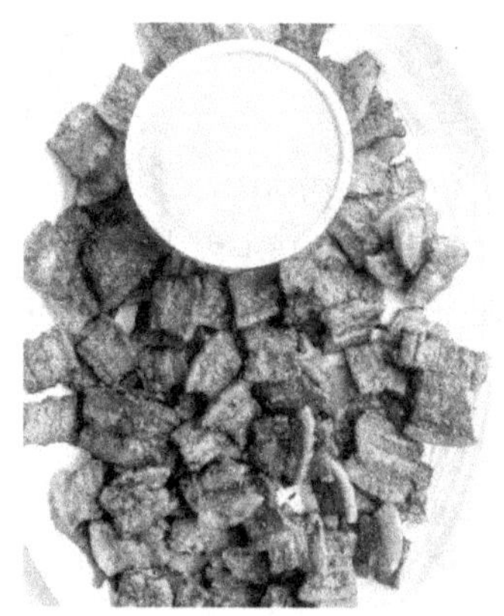

Table of Contents

Introduction

Welcome to "Carnivore Diet For Women Over 50," a transformative journey tailored specifically for women over 50 seeking optimal health and vitality. In this comprehensive guide, we delve into the fascinating world of the carnivore diet—a nutritional approach centered around animal-based foods—and explore its profound benefits for women in the prime of their lives.

As women age, hormonal fluctuations, metabolic changes, and shifting nutritional needs become paramount concerns. Traditional dietary recommendations often fall short in addressing these unique challenges, leaving many women feeling frustrated and deprived. However, the carnivore diet offers a refreshing paradigm shift, providing a simple yet powerful solution to reclaiming vibrant health and vitality.

Throughout this book, we will embark on a holistic exploration of the carnivore lifestyle, covering everything from its historical roots and scientific rationale to practical implementation strategies and meal planning tips specifically tailored for women over 50. We'll delve into the science behind why animal-based nutrition is uniquely suited to support female health in the later years, addressing common concerns such as bone health, muscle maintenance, hormonal balance, and cognitive function.

Prepare to unlock the full potential of your health and vitality as we embark on this transformative journey together. Let's embrace the carnivore lifestyle and thrive, not just survive, in the prime of our lives.

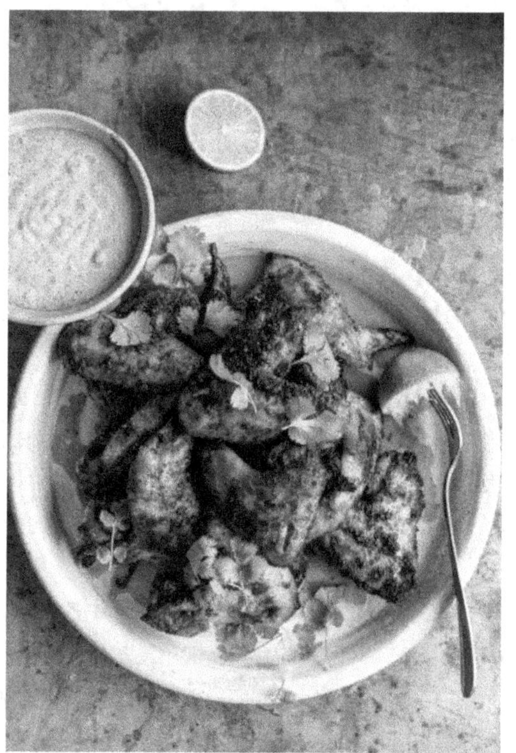

Benefits

1. Hormonal Balance: As women age, hormonal fluctuations become more pronounced, leading to issues such as menopause symptoms and imbalances. A carnivore diet can help stabilize hormone levels by providing essential nutrients like cholesterol, saturated fat, and amino acids necessary for hormone production.

2. Bone Health: Osteoporosis is a common concern for women as they age. Animal-based foods are rich in bioavailable nutrients like calcium, phosphorus, and vitamin D, essential for maintaining bone density and preventing fractures.

3. Muscle Maintenance: Sarcopenia, the loss of muscle mass and strength with age, can lead to mobility issues and decreased quality of life. The high-quality protein found in animal products supports muscle maintenance and repair, helping women over 50 stay strong and active.

4. Weight Management: Metabolic changes and decreased physical activity can make weight management challenging for women over 50. A carnivore diet, high in protein and low in carbohydrates, can support weight loss by promoting satiety, reducing cravings, and stabilizing blood sugar levels.

5. Mental Clarity: Cognitive function can decline with age, but a carnivore diet rich in nutrients like omega-3 fatty acids and B vitamins supports brain health, promoting mental clarity, focus, and memory retention.

6. Gut Health: Digestive issues become more prevalent as women age, but eliminating plant-based foods that may irritate the gut can alleviate symptoms like bloating, gas, and indigestion, promoting optimal digestive health.

By embracing a carnivore diet, women over 50 can experience improved hormonal balance, better bone health, enhanced muscle maintenance, effective weight management, sharper mental clarity, and improved gut health, empowering them to thrive in the later years of life.

Healthy Shopping Ingredients

1. Grass-fed Beef: Rich in protein, iron, and B vitamins, grass-fed beef is a staple of the carnivore diet, providing essential nutrients for muscle maintenance and overall health.

2. Pasture-Raised Eggs: A nutrient-dense source of protein, vitamins, and minerals, eggs are versatile and easy to incorporate into meals for added satiety and nutritional benefits.

3. Wild-Caught Fish: Salmon, mackerel, and sardines are excellent sources of omega-3 fatty acids, which support heart health, brain function, and inflammation reduction.

4. Organ Meats: Liver, kidney, and heart are nutrient powerhouses, packed with vitamins, minerals, and antioxidants essential for optimal health, including vitamin A, B vitamins, and iron.

5. Poultry: Chicken and turkey provide lean protein and essential nutrients like niacin and selenium, supporting muscle maintenance and immune function.

6. Bone Broth: Rich in collagen, gelatin, and amino acids, bone broth supports gut health, joint health, and skin elasticity, making it a valuable addition to the carnivore diet.

7. High-Quality Dairy: Full-fat dairy products like cheese and yogurt can be included in moderation for additional protein, calcium, and beneficial probiotics.

8. Bacon: A flavorful and satisfying addition to meals, bacon provides protein, fat, and essential nutrients, but choose varieties without added sugars or preservatives.

9. Lamb: Lamb is a nutrient-dense meat rich in protein, iron, and vitamin B12, supporting energy production, red blood cell formation, and immune function.

10. Beef Tallow: A stable cooking fat rich in saturated fats and fat-soluble vitamins, beef tallow adds flavor and nutrients to meals while supporting overall health.

11. Chicken Liver Pâté: A delicious and nutrient-dense spread, chicken liver pâté is high in vitamins A, D, E, and K, as well as iron and folate.

12. Shellfish: Shrimp, crab, and lobster provide protein, omega-3 fatty acids, and minerals like zinc and selenium, supporting immune function and overall health.

13. Duck: Duck is a flavorful and nutrient-rich meat high in protein, iron, and B vitamins, making it a valuable addition to the carnivore diet.

14. Beef Jerky: A convenient and portable snack, beef jerky provides protein and energy while satisfying hunger between meals, but opt for varieties without added sugars or preservatives.

15. Bone Marrow: Rich in healthy fats, collagen, and essential nutrients, bone marrow supports joint health, immune function, and skin elasticity.

16. Duck Eggs: Nutrient-dense alternatives to chicken eggs, duck eggs provide protein, vitamins, and minerals, offering variety and versatility in the carnivore diet.

17. Bison: Lean and flavorful, bison meat is high in protein, iron, and zinc, providing essential nutrients for muscle maintenance and overall health.

18. Pemmican: A traditional Native American food made from dried meat, fat, and berries, pemmican is a convenient and nutrient-dense snack for the carnivore diet.

19. Sardines in Olive Oil: A convenient source of omega-3 fatty acids, protein, and calcium, sardines in olive oil are a nutritious addition to the carnivore diet, supporting heart health, brain function, and bone density.

When shopping for a carnivore diet, prioritize high-quality, nutrient-dense animal products from sources such as grass-fed and pasture-raised animals, wild-caught fish, and organic options whenever possible to maximize health benefits.

Breakfast

1. Scrambled Eggs with Bacon

Ingredients:
- 3 large eggs
- 2 slices of bacon
- Salt and pepper to taste

Preparation:
1. Cook bacon in a skillet over medium heat until crispy. Remove and set aside.
2. In the same skillet, crack the eggs and scramble until cooked to desired consistency.
3. Season with salt and pepper.
4. Serve hot with crispy bacon on the side.

Nutritional Value:
- Calories: 350
- Protein: 22g
- Fat: 28g
- Cooking Time: 10 minutes

2. Egg and Cheese Omelette

Ingredients:
- 4 large eggs
- 1/4 cup shredded cheddar cheese
- Salt and pepper to taste

Preparation:

1. Crack the eggs into a bowl and whisk until well combined.

2. Heat a skillet over medium heat and pour the eggs into the pan.

3. Once the edges start to set, sprinkle the cheese over one half of the omelette.

4. Fold the other half of the omelette over the cheese and cook until the cheese is melted and the eggs are cooked through.

5. Season with salt and pepper.

6. Serve hot.

Nutritional Value:

- Calories: 360
- Protein: 26g
- Fat: 26g
- Cooking Time: 10 minutes

3. Steak and Eggs

Ingredients:

- 1 medium ribeye steak (8 oz)
- 2 large eggs
- Salt and pepper to taste

Preparation:

1. Season the steak with salt and pepper on both sides.

2. Heat a skillet over medium-high heat and cook the steak to desired doneness (about 4 minutes per side for medium-rare).

3. In the same skillet, cook the eggs sunny-side-up or to your preference.

4. Serve the steak with eggs on the side.

Nutritional Value:
  - Calories: 650
  - Protein: 56g
  - Fat: 45g
  - Cooking Time: 15 minutes

4. Bacon-Wrapped Sausages

Ingredients:
  - 4 pork sausages
  - 8 slices of bacon

Preparation:
1. Preheat the oven to 400°F (200°C).

2. Wrap each sausage with 2 slices of bacon, securing with toothpicks if necessary.

3. Place the bacon-wrapped sausages on a baking sheet lined with parchment paper.

4. Bake in the preheated oven for 20-25 minutes, or until the bacon is crispy and the sausages are cooked through.

5. Serve hot.

Nutritional Value:
- Calories: 500
- Protein: 32g
- Fat: 40g
- Cooking Time: 25 minutes

5. Salmon and Cream Cheese Roll-Ups

Ingredients:
- 4 slices of smoked salmon
- 4 tbsp cream cheese

Preparation:
1. Lay out the slices of smoked salmon on a clean surface.
2. Spread 1 tablespoon of cream cheese evenly over each slice.
3. Roll up the salmon slices tightly.
4. Slice each roll-up into bite-sized pieces.
5. Serve as is or with a side of scrambled eggs.

Nutritional Value:
- Calories: 280
- Protein: 20g
- Fat: 20g
- Cooking Time: 5 minutes

6. Egg Muffins with Ham and Cheese

Ingredients:
- 6 large eggs
- 1/2 cup diced ham
- 1/2 cup shredded cheddar cheese
- Salt and pepper to taste

Preparation:
1. Preheat the oven to 350°F (175°C) and grease a muffin tin.
2. In a bowl, whisk together the eggs, ham, cheese, salt, and pepper.
3. Pour the egg mixture into the prepared muffin tin, filling each cup about 3/4 full.
4. Bake in the preheated oven for 20-25 minutes, or until the egg muffins are set and golden brown.
5. Allow to cool slightly before serving.

Nutritional Value:
- Calories: 320
- Protein: 24g
- Fat: 22g
- Cooking Time: 25 minutes

7. Liver and Onions

Ingredients:
- 8 oz beef liver, sliced

- 1 large onion, sliced
- 2 tbsp butter or beef tallow
- Salt and pepper to taste

Preparation:

1. Heat the butter or beef tallow in a skillet over medium heat.

2. Add the sliced onions to the skillet and cook until caramelized, about 10 minutes.

3. Push the onions to the side of the skillet and add the sliced liver.

4. Cook the liver for 2-3 minutes per side, or until cooked through but still pink in the center.

5. Season with salt and pepper.

6. Serve hot with the caramelized onions on top.

Nutritional Value:

- Calories: 400
- Protein: 32g
- Fat: 26g
- Cooking Time: 15 minutes

8. Egg Drop Soup with Chicken

- Ingredients:
  - 4 cups chicken broth
  - 2 large eggs, beaten
  - 1 cup cooked chicken, shredded
  - Salt and pepper to taste

Preparation:

1. In a pot, bring the chicken broth to a simmer over medium heat.

2. Slowly pour the beaten eggs into the simmering broth while stirring gently to create ribbons of egg.

3. Add the shredded chicken to the soup and simmer for another 2-3 minutes.

4. Season with salt and pepper.

5. Serve hot.

Nutritional Value:
- Calories: 240
- Protein: 24g
- Fat: 10g
- Cooking Time: 10 minutes

9. Beef Bone Broth

Ingredients:
- 2 lbs beef bones (marrow bones or knuckle bones)
- 2 carrots, chopped
- 2 celery stalks, chopped
- 1 onion, quartered
- 4 cloves garlic, smashed
- 2 bay leaves
- Salt and pepper to taste
- Water

Preparation:

1. Preheat the oven to 400°F (200°C).

2. Place the beef bones on a baking sheet and roast in the preheated oven for 30 minutes, or until browned.

3. Transfer the roasted bones to a large pot and add the chopped vegetables, garlic, bay leaves, salt, and pepper.

4. Fill the pot with enough water to cover the bones and vegetables.

5. Bring the mixture to a boil, then reduce the heat to low and simmer, uncovered, for 8-10 hours, skimming any foam that rises to the surface.

6. Strain the broth through a fine-mesh sieve or cheesecloth and discard the solids.

7. Allow the broth to cool before storing in the refrigerator or freezer.

8. Reheat before serving.

Nutritional Value (per cup):

- Calories: 50
- Protein: 5g
- Fat: 3g
- Cooking Time: 10 hours

10. Beef Liver Pâté

- Ingredients:
  - 1 lb beef liver, sliced
  - 1 onion, chopped
  - 2 cloves garlic, minced

- 1/2 cup beef tallow
- Salt and pepper to taste

Preparation:

1. In a skillet, heat 2 tablespoons of beef tallow over medium heat.

2. Add the chopped onion and minced garlic to the skillet and cook until softened, about 5 minutes.

3. Push the onions and garlic to the side of the skillet and add the sliced liver.

4. Cook the liver for 2-3 minutes per side, or until cooked through but still pink in the center.

5. Transfer the cooked liver, onions, and garlic to a food processor and add the remaining beef tallow.

6. Process until smooth, then season with salt and pepper to taste.

7. Transfer the pâté to a container and refrigerate until firm.

8. Serve chilled with sliced cucumber or celery.

Nutritional Value (per tablespoon):

- Calories: 50
- Protein: 4g
- Fat: 3g
- Cooking Time: 15 minutes

These recipes offer a variety of options for delicious and nutritious breakfasts tailored to the carnivore diet, providing ample protein, healthy fats, and essential nutrients to support

23 Carnivore Diet For Women Over 50

women over 50 in maintaining optimal health and vitality. Adjust ingredients and quantities as needed to suit individual preferences and dietary requirements.

Lunch

1. Beef and Bacon Lettuce Wraps

Ingredients:
- 8 oz ground beef
- 4 slices bacon
- Large lettuce leaves
- Salt and pepper to taste

Preparation:
1. Cook bacon in a skillet until crispy. Remove and set aside.
2. In the same skillet, cook ground beef until browned and cooked through. Season with salt and pepper.
3. Place a spoonful of cooked ground beef onto each lettuce leaf.
4. Crumble bacon on top.
5. Wrap the lettuce leaves around the filling.
6. Serve immediately.

Nutritional Value (per serving):
- Calories: 400
- Protein: 30g
- Fat: 30g
- Cooking Time: 15 minutes

2. Salmon Patties

- Ingredients:
  - 2 cans (6 oz each) of canned salmon, drained
  - 2 eggs
  - Salt and pepper to taste
  - 2 tbsp butter or beef tallow

Preparation:

1. In a bowl, mix together drained salmon, eggs, salt, and pepper until well combined.
2. Form the mixture into patties.
3. Heat butter or beef tallow in a skillet over medium heat.
4. Cook the salmon patties for 3-4 minutes on each side, or until golden brown and cooked through.
5. Serve hot.

Nutritional Value (per serving):
- Calories: 350
- Protein: 40g
- Fat: 20g
- Cooking Time: 10 minutes

3. Beef and Cheese Roll-Ups

Ingredients:
- 8 slices roast beef
- 4 slices cheddar cheese
- Salt and pepper to taste

Preparation:
1. Lay out the slices of roast beef on a clean surface.
2. Place a slice of cheese on each slice of roast beef.
3. Roll up tightly.
4. Season with salt and pepper if desired.
5. Serve as is or with a side of mustard or horseradish.

Nutritional Value (per serving):
- Calories: 450
- Protein: 40g
- Fat: 30g
- Cooking Time: 5 minutes

4. Chicken Caesar Salad

- Ingredients:
  - 8 oz cooked chicken breast, sliced
  - Romaine lettuce, chopped
  - Caesar dressing (check for sugar-free options)
  - Parmesan cheese, grated
  - Salt and pepper to taste

- Preparation:
  1. Place chopped romaine lettuce in a bowl.
  2. Top with sliced cooked chicken breast.
  3. Drizzle with Caesar dressing.
  4. Sprinkle with grated Parmesan cheese.
  5. Season with salt and pepper.
  6. Toss to combine.

7. Serve immediately.

- Nutritional Value (per serving):
  - Calories: 400
  - Protein: 40g
  - Fat: 20g
  - Cooking Time: 15 minutes

5. Beef Liver Stir-Fry

Ingredients:
- 8 oz beef liver, thinly sliced
- 1 onion, sliced
- 1 bell pepper, sliced
- 2 tbsp butter or beef tallow
- Salt and pepper to taste

Preparation:
1. Heat butter or beef tallow in a skillet over medium heat.
2. Add sliced onion and bell pepper to the skillet and cook until softened.
3. Push the vegetables to the side and add the sliced beef liver to the skillet.
4. Cook the liver for 2-3 minutes per side, or until cooked through but still pink in the center.
5. Season with salt and pepper.
6. Serve hot.

Nutritional Value (per serving):
- Calories: 350
- Protein: 30g
- Fat: 20g
- Cooking Time: 15 minutes

6. Bison Burger Salad

Ingredients:
- 8 oz bison burger patty
- Mixed salad greens
- Ranch dressing (check for sugar-free options)
- Salt and pepper to taste

Preparation:
1. Cook bison burger patty on a grill or skillet until cooked to desired doneness.
2. Place mixed salad greens on a plate.
3. Top with cooked bison burger patty.
4. Drizzle with ranch dressing.
5. Season with salt and pepper.
6. Serve immediately.

Nutritional Value (per serving):
- Calories: 450
- Protein: 40g
- Fat: 30g
- Cooking Time: 10 minutes

Ingredients:
- 4 hard-boiled eggs, chopped
- 2 tbsp mayonnaise (check for sugar-free options)
- Salt and pepper to taste
- Large lettuce leaves

Preparation:
1. In a bowl, mix together chopped hard-boiled eggs, mayonnaise, salt, and pepper until well combined.
2. Place a spoonful of egg salad onto each lettuce leaf.
3. Wrap the lettuce leaves around the filling.
4. Serve immediately.

Nutritional Value (per serving):
- Calories: 300
- Protein: 20g
- Fat: 25g
- Cooking Time: 10 minutes

8. Shrimp Scampi

- Ingredients:
- 8 oz shrimp, peeled and deveined
- 2 cloves garlic, minced
- 2 tbsp butter
- Salt and pepper to taste

Preparation:

1. Heat butter in a skillet over medium heat.

2. Add minced garlic to the skillet and cook until fragrant.

3. Add shrimp to the skillet and cook for 2-3 minutes per side, or until pink and cooked through.

4. Season with salt and pepper.

5. Serve hot.

Nutritional Value (per serving):

- Calories: 300
- Protein: 25g
- Fat: 15g
- Cooking Time: 10 minutes

9. Beef Bone Broth Soup

Ingredients:

- 4 cups beef bone broth
- 8 oz cooked beef, shredded or diced
- Salt and pepper to taste

Preparation:

1. In a pot, bring beef bone broth to a simmer over medium heat.

2. Add cooked beef to the pot and simmer for 5-10 minutes, or until heated through.

3. Season with salt and pepper.

4. Serve hot.

Nutritional Value (per serving):
- Calories: 250
- Protein: 20g
- Fat: 15g
- Cooking Time: 10 minutes

10. Turkey and Cheese Roll-Ups

Ingredients:
- 8 slices deli turkey
- 4 slices cheese (cheddar, Swiss, or your choice)
- Salt and pepper to taste

Preparation:
1. Lay out the slices of deli turkey on a clean surface.
2. Place a slice of cheese on each slice of turkey.
3. Roll up tightly.
4. Season with salt and pepper if desired.
5. Serve as is or with a side of mustard or mayonnaise.

Nutritional Value (per serving):
- Calories: 350
- Protein: 30g
- Fat: 20g
- Cooking Time: 5 minutes

These lunch recipes provide a variety of delicious options for women over 50 following a carnivore diet, offering ample protein, healthy fats, and essential nutrients to support optimal health and well-being. Adjust ingredients and quantities as needed to suit individual preferences and dietary requirements.

Dinner

1. Ribeye Steak with Garlic Butter

Ingredients:
- 1 ribeye steak (8 oz)
- 2 tbsp butter
- 2 cloves garlic, minced
- Salt and pepper to taste

Preparation:
1. Season the ribeye steak with salt and pepper on both sides.
2. Heat a skillet over medium-high heat and cook the steak to desired doneness (about 4 minutes per side for medium-rare).
3. In a small saucepan, melt the butter over low heat.
4. Add minced garlic to the melted butter and cook for 1-2 minutes until fragrant.
5. Pour garlic butter over the cooked steak before serving.

Nutritional Value (per serving):
- Calories: 600
- Protein: 50g
- Fat: 45g
- Cooking Time: 10 minutes

2. Bacon-Wrapped Filet Mignon

Ingredients:
- 2 filet mignon steaks (6 oz each)
- 4 slices bacon
- Salt and pepper to taste

Preparation:
1. Preheat the oven to 400°F (200°C).
2. Season the filet mignon steaks with salt and pepper on both sides.
3. Wrap each steak with 2 slices of bacon, securing with toothpicks if necessary.
4. Place the wrapped steaks on a baking sheet lined with parchment paper.
5. Bake in the preheated oven for 20-25 minutes, or until the bacon is crispy and the steaks are cooked to desired doneness.
6. Remove toothpicks before serving.

Nutritional Value (per serving):
- Calories: 600
- Protein: 50g
- Fat: 40g
- Cooking Time: 25 minutes

3. Grilled Salmon with Lemon Butter Sauce

Ingredients:
- 2 salmon fillets (6 oz each)
- 2 tbsp butter
- Juice of 1 lemon
- Salt and pepper to taste

Preparation:
1. Preheat the grill to medium-high heat.
2. Season the salmon fillets with salt and pepper.
3. Grill the salmon fillets for 4-5 minutes per side, or until cooked through and flaky.
4. In a small saucepan, melt the butter over low heat.
5. Add lemon juice to the melted butter and stir to combine.
6. Pour lemon butter sauce over the grilled salmon before serving.

Nutritional Value (per serving):
- Calories: 450
- Protein: 40g
- Fat: 30g
- Cooking Time: 10 minutes

4. Beef Short Ribs

Ingredients:
- 2 lbs beef short ribs

- Salt and pepper to taste

Preparation:
1. Preheat the oven to 300°F (150°C).
2. Season the beef short ribs with salt and pepper on all sides.
3. Place the ribs in a roasting pan or baking dish.
4. Cover with foil and bake in the preheated oven for 3-4 hours, or until the meat is tender and falling off the bone.
5. Remove foil and broil for 2-3 minutes to crisp up the edges if desired.
6. Serve hot.

Nutritional Value (per serving):
- Calories: 800
- Protein: 60g
- Fat: 60g
- Cooking Time: 3-4 hours

5. Chicken Thighs with Herbs

Ingredients:
- 4 chicken thighs, bone-in and skin-on
- 2 tbsp olive oil
- 2 tsp dried herbs (such as thyme, rosemary, or oregano)
- Salt and pepper to taste

Preparation:
1. Preheat the oven to 400°F (200°C).

2. Rub chicken thighs with olive oil and season with dried herbs, salt, and pepper.

3. Place the seasoned chicken thighs on a baking sheet lined with parchment paper.

4. Bake in the preheated oven for 30-35 minutes, or until the chicken is cooked through and the skin is crispy.

5. Serve hot.

Nutritional Value (per serving):
- Calories: 450
- Protein: 40g
- Fat: 30g
- Cooking Time: 35 minutes

6. Beef Liver and Onions

Ingredients:
- 1 lb beef liver, sliced
- 2 large onions, sliced
- 2 tbsp butter or beef tallow
- Salt and pepper to taste

Preparation:
1. Heat butter or beef tallow in a skillet over medium heat.

2. Add sliced onions to the skillet and cook until caramelized, about 10 minutes.

3. Push the onions to the side of the skillet and add the sliced beef liver.

4. Cook the liver for 2-3 minutes per side, or until cooked through but still pink in the center.

5. Season with salt and pepper.

6. Serve hot with caramelized onions on top.

Nutritional Value (per serving):
- Calories: 400
- Protein: 30g
- Fat: 25g
- Cooking Time: 15 minutes

7. Lamb Chops with Mint Sauce

Ingredients:
- 4 lamb chops
- 2 tbsp olive oil
- 2 tbsp fresh mint, chopped
- Salt and pepper to taste

Preparation:
1. Preheat the grill to medium-high heat.

2. Rub lamb chops with olive oil and season with salt and pepper.

3. Grill lamb chops for 3-4 minutes per side for medium-rare, or until desired doneness.

4. In a small bowl, mix chopped mint with a pinch of salt.

5. Serve grilled lamb chops with mint sauce on top.

Nutritional Value (per serving):
    - Calories: 600
    - Protein: 50g
    - Fat: 40g
    - Cooking Time: 10 minutes

8. Beef Bacon-Wrapped Asparagus

Ingredients:
    - 1 lb asparagus spears, trimmed
    - 8 slices beef bacon
    - Salt and pepper to taste

Preparation:
    1. Preheat the oven to 400°F (200°C).
    2. Wrap each asparagus spear with a slice of beef bacon.
    3. Place the wrapped asparagus spears on a baking sheet lined with parchment paper.
    4. Bake in the preheated oven for 15-20 minutes, or until the bacon is crispy and the asparagus is tender.
    5. Season with salt and pepper.
    6. Serve hot.

Nutritional Value (per serving):
    - Calories: 300
    - Protein: 20g
    - Fat: 25g
    - Cooking Time: 20 minutes

9. Turkey Meatballs

Ingredients:
- 1 lb ground turkey
- 1 egg
- 1/4 cup almond flour
- 2 cloves garlic, minced
- Salt and pepper to taste

Preparation:
1. Preheat the oven to 400°F (200°C).
2. In a bowl, mix together ground turkey, egg, almond flour, minced garlic, salt, and pepper until well combined.
3. Form the mixture into meatballs and place them on a baking sheet lined with parchment paper.
4. Bake in the preheated oven for 20-25 minutes, or until the meatballs are cooked through.
5. Serve hot with your favorite dipping sauce or gravy.

Nutritional Value (per serving):
- Calories: 350
- Protein: 30g
- Fat: 20g
- Cooking Time: 25 minutes

10. Beef Stir-Fry with Vegetables

Ingredients:
- 1 lb beef steak, thinly sliced

- 2 cups mixed vegetables (such as bell peppers, broccoli, and mushrooms)
- 2 tbsp beef tallow
- Salt and pepper to taste

Preparation:
1. Heat beef tallow in a skillet or wok over high heat.
2. Add sliced beef to the skillet and stir-fry for 2-3 minutes, or until browned.
3. Add mixed vegetables to the skillet and continue to stir-fry for another 3-4 minutes, or until vegetables are tender-crisp.
4. Season with salt and pepper.
5. Serve hot.

Nutritional Value (per serving):
- Calories: 500
- Protein: 40g
- Fat: 35g
- Cooking Time: 10 minutes

These dinner recipes provide a variety of delicious options for women over 50 following a carnivore diet, offering ample protein, healthy fats, and essential nutrients to support optimal health and well-being. Adjust ingredients and quantities as needed to suit individual preferences and dietary requirements.

Snacks

1. Bacon-Wrapped Jalapeño Poppers

Ingredients:
- 6 jalapeño peppers, halved and seeds removed
- 6 slices bacon, cut in half

Preparation:
1. Preheat the oven to 400°F (200°C).
2. Stuff each jalapeño half with cream cheese.
3. Wrap each stuffed jalapeño half with a half slice of bacon.
4. Place the wrapped jalapeños on a baking sheet lined with parchment paper.
5. Bake in the preheated oven for 20-25 minutes, or until the bacon is crispy.
6. Serve hot.

Nutritional Value (per serving, 3 poppers):
- Calories: 250
- Protein: 10g
- Fat: 20g
- Cooking Time: 25 minutes

2. Beef Jerky

- Ingredients:
- 1 lb beef steak (such as flank or sirloin), thinly sliced

- 1/4 cup soy sauce or coconut aminos
- 1 tbsp Worcestershire sauce (optional)
- 1 tsp garlic powder
- 1 tsp onion powder
- 1/2 tsp black pepper

Preparation:

1. In a bowl, mix together soy sauce, Worcestershire sauce (if using), garlic powder, onion powder, and black pepper.

2. Add thinly sliced beef to the marinade and toss to coat evenly.

3. Cover and refrigerate for at least 2 hours, or overnight.

4. Preheat the oven to 175°F (80°C) or the lowest setting.

5. Place marinated beef slices on a baking sheet lined with parchment paper.

6. Bake in the preheated oven for 4-6 hours, or until the beef is dried and chewy.

7. Let cool before serving.

Nutritional Value (per serving, 2 oz):
- Calories: 200
- Protein: 20g
- Fat: 10g
- Cooking Time: 4-6 hours

3. Egg Salad

Ingredients:
- 4 hard-boiled eggs, chopped
- 2 tbsp mayonnaise (check for sugar-free options)
- Salt and pepper to taste

Preparation:
1. In a bowl, mix together chopped hard-boiled eggs and mayonnaise until well combined.
2. Season with salt and pepper to taste.
3. Serve chilled.

Nutritional Value (per serving, 1/2 cup):
- Calories: 250
- Protein: 15g
- Fat: 20g
- Cooking Time: 10 minutes

4. Smoked Salmon Roll-Ups

Ingredients:
- 4 slices smoked salmon
- 4 tbsp cream cheese
- 2 tbsp chopped chives or dill (optional)

Preparation:
1. Lay out the slices of smoked salmon on a clean surface.

2. Spread 1 tablespoon of cream cheese evenly over each slice.

3. Sprinkle chopped chives or dill over the cream cheese, if using.

4. Roll up the salmon slices tightly.

5. Slice each roll-up into bite-sized pieces.

6. Serve chilled.

Nutritional Value (per serving, 2 roll-ups):
- Calories: 150
- Protein: 10g
- Fat: 10g
- Cooking Time: 5 minutes

5. Beef Bone Broth

Ingredients:
- 2 lbs beef bones (marrow bones or knuckle bones)
- 2 carrots, chopped
- 2 celery stalks, chopped
- 1 onion, quartered
- 4 cloves garlic, smashed
- 2 bay leaves
- Salt and pepper to taste
- Water

Preparation:
1. Preheat the oven to 400°F (200°C).

2. Place the beef bones on a baking sheet and roast in the preheated oven for 30 minutes, or until browned.

3. Transfer the roasted bones to a large pot and add the chopped vegetables, garlic, bay leaves, salt, and pepper.

4. Fill the pot with enough water to cover the bones and vegetables.

5. Bring the mixture to a boil, then reduce the heat to low and simmer, uncovered, for 8-10 hours, skimming any foam that rises to the surface.

6. Strain the broth through a fine-mesh sieve or cheesecloth and discard the solids.

7. Allow the broth to cool before storing in the refrigerator or freezer.

8. Reheat before serving.

Nutritional Value (per cup):
- Calories: 50
- Protein: 5g
- Fat: 3g
- Cooking Time: 10 hours

These snack recipes offer a variety of delicious options for women over 50 following a carnivore diet, providing ample protein, healthy fats, and essential nutrients to support optimal health and well-being. Adjust ingredients and quantities as needed to suit individual preferences and dietary requirements.

Conclusion

The carnivore diet offers women over 50 a promising approach to enhance their health and well-being. Through its emphasis on high-quality animal-based foods, this dietary regimen provides essential nutrients such as protein, vitamins, and minerals, which are crucial for supporting muscle strength, bone density, and overall vitality. By eliminating processed foods, grains, and sugars, the carnivore diet can help regulate blood sugar levels, reduce inflammation, and promote weight management, thereby mitigating the risk of chronic diseases such as diabetes, heart disease, and obesity.

Furthermore, the simplicity and versatility of carnivore diet recipes make it accessible and practical for women over 50 to incorporate into their lifestyles. With a wide range of delicious meal options, including steaks, seafood, and nutrient-rich organ meats, adhering to this dietary approach can be both satisfying and enjoyable.

As women over 50 navigate the complexities of aging and strive to maintain their health and vitality, the carnivore diet stands out as a viable solution. By prioritizing nutrient-dense animal foods and minimizing dietary toxins, individuals can optimize their nutrition and support their bodies' natural healing processes.

In adopting and adapting to the carnivore diet, women over 50 have the opportunity to reclaim their health, enhance their quality of life, and embrace a lifestyle rooted in simplicity and nourishment. With dedication and perseverance, each meal becomes an opportunity to nourish the body and cultivate a stronger, more resilient self. Embrace the carnivore diet not just as a dietary choice, but as a pathway to empowerment and well-being. Your body deserves the best, and the carnivore diet offers a path towards achieving it.

Bonus

Unlock the full potential of your new favorite cookbook with our paperback edition, now featuring an exclusive meal planner bonus! Dive into delicious recipes while effortlessly organizing your weekly meals. Enjoy the convenience and practicality of having everything you need at your fingertips. Upgrade to the paperback today!

Weekly Meal Planner

Monday

Breakfast	
Lunch	
Dinner	

Tuesday

Breakfast	
Lunch	
Dinner	

Wednesday

Breakfast	
Lunch	
Dinner	

Thursday

Breakfast	
Lunch	
Dinner	

Friday

Breakfast	
Lunch	
Dinner	

Saturday

Breakfast	
Lunch	
Dinner	

Sunday

Breakfast	
Lunch	
Dinner	

Noted

Weekly Meal Planner

Monday

Breakfast	
Lunch	
Dinner	

Tuesday

Breakfast	
Lunch	
Dinner	

Wednesday

Breakfast	
Lunch	
Dinner	

Thursday

Breakfast	
Lunch	
Dinner	

Friday

Breakfast	
Lunch	
Dinner	

Saturday

Breakfast	
Lunch	
Dinner	

Sunday

Breakfast	
Lunch	
Dinner	

Noted

Weekly Meal Planner

Monday

Breakfast	
Lunch	
Dinner	

Tuesday

Breakfast	
Lunch	
Dinner	

Wednesday

Breakfast	
Lunch	
Dinner	

Thursday

Breakfast	
Lunch	
Dinner	

Friday

Breakfast	
Lunch	
Dinner	

Saturday

Breakfast	
Lunch	
Dinner	

Sunday

Breakfast	
Lunch	
Dinner	

Noted

Weekly Meal Planner

Monday

Breakfast	
Lunch	
Dinner	

Tuesday

Breakfast	
Lunch	
Dinner	

Wednesday

Breakfast	
Lunch	
Dinner	

Thursday

Breakfast	
Lunch	
Dinner	

Friday

Breakfast	
Lunch	
Dinner	

Saturday

Breakfast	
Lunch	
Dinner	

Sunday

Breakfast	
Lunch	
Dinner	

Noted

Weekly Meal Planner

Monday

Breakfast	
Lunch	
Dinner	

Tuesday

Breakfast	
Lunch	
Dinner	

Wednesday

Breakfast	
Lunch	
Dinner	

Thursday

Breakfast	
Lunch	
Dinner	

Friday

Breakfast	
Lunch	
Dinner	

Saturday

Breakfast	
Lunch	
Dinner	

Sunday

Breakfast	
Lunch	
Dinner	

Noted

Weekly Meal Planner

Monday

Breakfast	
Lunch	
Dinner	

Tuesday

Breakfast	
Lunch	
Dinner	

Wednesday

Breakfast	
Lunch	
Dinner	

Thursday

Breakfast	
Lunch	
Dinner	

Friday

Breakfast	
Lunch	
Dinner	

Saturday

Breakfast	
Lunch	
Dinner	

Sunday

Breakfast	
Lunch	
Dinner	

Noted

Weekly Meal Planner

Monday

Breakfast	
Lunch	
Dinner	

Tuesday

Breakfast	
Lunch	
Dinner	

Wednesday

Breakfast	
Lunch	
Dinner	

Thursday

Breakfast	
Lunch	
Dinner	

Friday

Breakfast	
Lunch	
Dinner	

Saturday

Breakfast	
Lunch	
Dinner	

Sunday

Breakfast	
Lunch	
Dinner	

Noted

Weekly Meal Planner

Monday

Breakfast	
Lunch	
Dinner	

Tuesday

Breakfast	
Lunch	
Dinner	

Wednesday

Breakfast	
Lunch	
Dinner	

Thursday

Breakfast	
Lunch	
Dinner	

Friday

Breakfast	
Lunch	
Dinner	

Saturday

Breakfast	
Lunch	
Dinner	

Sunday

Breakfast	
Lunch	
Dinner	

Noted

Weekly Meal Planner

Monday

Breakfast	
Lunch	
Dinner	

Tuesday

Breakfast	
Lunch	
Dinner	

Wednesday

Breakfast	
Lunch	
Dinner	

Thursday

Breakfast	
Lunch	
Dinner	

Friday

Breakfast	
Lunch	
Dinner	

Saturday

Breakfast	
Lunch	
Dinner	

Sunday

Breakfast	
Lunch	
Dinner	

Noted

Weekly Meal Planner

Monday

Breakfast	
Lunch	
Dinner	

Tuesday

Breakfast	
Lunch	
Dinner	

Wednesday

Breakfast	
Lunch	
Dinner	

Thursday

Breakfast	
Lunch	
Dinner	

Friday

Breakfast	
Lunch	
Dinner	

Saturday

Breakfast	
Lunch	
Dinner	

Sunday

Breakfast	
Lunch	
Dinner	

Noted